Nutrition for Special Needs

What shall I feed my Child?

Sue Cook and Karen Stevenson

ISBN:1516898672
ISBN-13: 9781516898671

Dedication

I dedicate this book to my family. My mother Rosemary Redfern for discovering that my father had food intolerances. To my father Mick Ford for going with Mum's help and being brave enough to make changes. To them both for inspiring me and educating me. To my sons Toby and Stefan who have accompanied me on this journey and been brilliant fun and a joy.
Sue Cook

CONTENTS

Free Chapters from my other books:

Lefthanders;

Being dyscalculate

ACKNOWLEDGMENTS

To Sally Bunday who developed the Hyperactive Children Support Group in the seventies and helped my father so much over the years. To Svea Gold my teacher, who encouraged me to learn neurodevelopment. To all the people who have allowed me to help them recover their health.
Sue Cook

How it all Started
1

Back in the seventies my father, now 80, (the one who trained as a dyslexia teacher when he retired), used to suffer from terrible migraines that would put him in bed for three days.

By chance my mother heard a radio programme about food additives. The woman being interviewed had just started the hyperactive children's support group (HACSG) to help her son and other children like him.

My father contacted the group, cured his headaches, and started helping other parents with hyperactive children in our area. He does still does it now thirty years later.

During this time, I too have learnt what they have to say, put it into practice with countless people over the years, and helped relieve suffering in the process.

This book will guide you through the maze of potential health disasters drawing on almost thirty years of my experience with foods as well my nutrition training at university. My good friend Karen Stevenson who trained with me at university and is also a qualified Nutritional Therapist.

So how does what we eat affect our ability to read? I can hear you asking.

Nutrients from our food provide the building blocks for the growth, repair and replacement of all the cells in the body, including those in the brain. If we don't take in the right nutrients, we can't build healthy cells and without healthy cells we don't have a healthy body or brain.

Worse still, if the food we eat contains unnatural, potentially harmful compounds, these can not only push out the beneficial nutrients but may even damage the cells in our bodies and seriously sabotage our health.

If there is not enough of the right nutrients in our diets, important functions in the body do not work as well as they should. At the extreme end of nutrient deficiency we could develop for example, diseases such as rickets, or scurvy. Everybody now knows what causes these conditions, and these days they are largely avoided in first world countries thanks to governments recognising and establishing Recommended Daily Allowances (RDAs).

1.1 RDAs

RDAs are the amount of each nutrient a person should consume on a daily basis. Unfortunately however, RDAs have for a long time now been considered to be the bare minimum level of nutrients required to keep deficiency diseases at bay. They are not anywhere near sufficient to maintain optimum health or optimum brain function.

RDAs have been set to ensure that the general population do not suffer from deficiency diseases; they do not take account of individual needs which can vary from person to person and over time in the same person. Our individual nutrient needs may be higher due to genetic variations, the quality of our diets, our level of physical activity, infections, illness, and even the level of stress in our lives.

1.2 Deficiency

Also, not all nutrients have an RDA. So, in addition to many of the RDAs being set too low for optimum health, some important nutrients are often forgotten about all together.

Karen says: Young and old can still suffer from vitamin and mineral deficiencies but nowadays in Western societies it tends to be more at a subclinical level. That means it is not at such an extreme level that obvious deficiency signs and symptoms are apparent, although in some cases there is, but that milder symptoms of poor health exist and remain persistent. Often by increasing some or all of the vital nutrients needed for good health, symptoms improve and a better level of health and functioning is achieved.

There are many deficiencies going on today that people do not know about, or do know and ignore. I will explain why it is absolutely important to take this information seriously.

There are many people including children walking round today with the modern equivalent of scurvy because they refuse to believe that their food is making them ill.

It is not right that our young, and our adults for that matter, are never without a cold, or the sniffs.

Our young should be radiating vitality and have a clear head and enthusiasm.

I will tell you how to work towards achieving that goal. It is cheaper, healthier and more rewarding to be eating food that is nurturing you not harming you.

1.3 Concentration

Karen says: the type of food we eat can also affect our energy levels, which in turn can affect our level of concentration. Your child needs to be able to concentrate in order to learn.

It's also not all about what you eat that can affect your child's ability to read, write and learn.

It's also about when you eat. Skipping meals can play havoc with energy levels and your child's ability to concentrate. Our brains not only need a constant supply of the right nutrients for it to develop and remain healthy, it also needs a constant supply of fuel to function properly. I will talk more about this later.

1.4 Food Reactions

Over the years that I have been in practice I have seen many, many health issues resolved by a change in diet. These were illnesses that the patient had had for years and had tried everything to no avail.

So when they got to me they were desperate and in pain.

In one case a woman had swollen feet that oozed puss out of the toenails, the skin was flaky and her feet were sore. I discovered that this was an egg allergy and after not eating eggs the symptoms resolved.

In another case a young lad had red raised trails all over his arms that looked like a creature had been burrowing along. He had seen a skin specialist and no one knew what was wrong. He came to me and I worked out that it was a reaction to tomatoes. He was eating loads of them, and the skin condition resolved quickly when he stopped eating tomatoes.

Nutrition for Special Needs

A young child of ten years old came to see me with a sore tongue. I soon discovered that he was eating loads of sugar free gum. The artificial sweeteners used in these products are well known to cause tongue sensitivity. He refused the give up the gum, so I expect he still has a sore tongue.

In cases like these, there was one cause and it was easy enough to work out. But not all health issues are straightforward. And when we have learning disorders, there could be many contributing factors. So this book will address things you can easily do at home.

I know from experience that suggesting to people that they change their diet is like asking them to donate a kidney.

And actually getting people to change the way they do things is like trying to put an octopus in a string bag. Getting children to eat vegetables and less sugar is like trying to push a jelly uphill. IT IS TEDIOUS AND FRUSTRATING, but unlike the jelly situation it is very important.

I know it is hard, I wouldn't suggest you do anything I don't do or haven't done.

I have even had someone say to me that burgers from a famous company are very good food, after all it is only bread, meat and a few bits of lettuce, so what can be the problem?

If this has been your attitude then we have a lot of work to do to educate you about food. For a start that kind of food is loaded with saturated fats and sugar, and is very highly processed. It is unhealthy.

The most willing people, I find, to change their diets, are those that have had health problems.

What motivation is there for people who eat any old rubbish and seem healthy enough? Not much, except that ten years later they have developed diabetes or had a heart attack like two of our friends.

These two chaps were built like oxen and ate whatever they wanted, drank loads of alcohol and punished their bodies, ignoring the signs. Now, one developed very serious diabetes in his mid thirties and had to give up his very successful career, and the other is recovering from a heart attack at the age of 42. The choice is yours. Health is precious, look after it.

Elimination Diets

2

I expect you are wondering what foods made my father have those migraines back in the seventies and how that links in with hyperactive children.

He eliminated certain foods that typically cause reactions including chocolate, nuts, cheese, monosodium glutamate, colourings, flavourings, preservatives, flavour enhancers, sodium nitrate, and sodium nitrite. After some time he carefully reintroduced certain foods and found that he reacted to monosodium glutamate, and the worst offenders were nitrates which actually make him unable to stand and he can hallucinate from them.

These foods mentioned that he eliminated for a time, are often the culprits with children along with sensitivity to oranges.

Now, there are two sides to this. One is that people can react to these foods and the other is that if they are deficient in, say, essential fatty acids, then they are more likely to have reactions.

So, the process of getting well involves taking out the things that don't suit and putting in things where deficiency might be.

I will give you general advice that most people would benefit from, but there will be individuals who have needs outside this and for that you need tailor made care from a nutritional therapist.

This book will bring most people up to a level within which they should be able to function a lot better than they were. For many an improved diet can bring about dramatic changes.

I aim to give you practical, doable solutions in this book that will explain and educate you so that soon you do have happy, healthy children.

2.1 Chronic fatigue

Now before you think I am going to go all preachy on you, you might be surprised to learn that even though I knew all this stuff from a young age, when I got my first house at 20, I would eat anything, drink anything, and I was not very discerning about the quality of what I ate.

I was recovering from the most severe case of glandular fever that had nearly killed me, aged 19, and my periods had stopped. I suffered with frequent colds and joint pains. I also had severe post viral fatigue syndrome.

I was partying all the time and drinking alcohol on a regular basis, staying up late and not exercising at all.

A friend who was a Chinese Herbalist visited me one day and he was shocked by what I was eating. 'That is dead food with no nutritional content at all, do you want to be ill?' he asked me.

Well no, I did not want to be ill. I wanted to feel great and be bursting with vitality. It was certainly food for thought. I realised if he was right, then that was why I was ill, and not recovering.

I wanted health, I wanted to feel well. I had already realised that health was not something to take for granted. It was a treasure to be nurtured.

So I gradually began reading more books on nutrition and health. I realised that health was probably the most important ingredient we had in life. Without it, we are nothing.

I learnt things that challenged many of the 'facts' I had been told about food such as milk being good for us. Milk is calf food, full of hormones to help them grow into great big cows and is way too rich for humans. Once we are weaned, us mammals do not require milk, especially that from another species. More on that later.

The Brain
3

So let's start with the brain.

Although the brain represents only 2% of the body's weight, it gets a whopping 20% of the body's blood flow. This is because blood carries oxygen, nutrients and glucose (the fuel for energy) to enable the brain to function effectively. The brain uses up an enormous amount of these substances and should any of them be in low supply it will begin to underfunction.

The brain starts developing in the womb but continues to grow for almost another 18 years. The brain is basically a network of special nerve cells called neurons. There are about 100 billion neurons in our brain and they communicate with each other by chemical messengers called neurotransmitters. I'll tell you more about these in a little while.

3.1 Neurons

As neurons communicate with each other, pathways become established in the brain, a bit like a road map, which is the basis for learning and memory.

Provided the right nutrients are in supply humans continue to make new neurons and their chemical messengers throughout life in response to mental activity, so it is never too late to train your brain.

3.2 Brain composition

Our brains are composed almost entirely of fat with a large percentage of water, and some protein. The type of fat we have in our diet therefore has a big influence on the type of fat that gets incorporated into the brain.

But it's not just any old fat that makes for a sharp, healthy and happy brain. The best fats for making a healthy brain are what are commonly known as essential fats.

3.3 Essential fats

These are a vital type of food that often tends to get left out of people's diets due to a fear of getting fat but they really are essential in every way. Our bodies cannot make them, so we have to eat them.

Not all fats found in food actually make you fat! Some fats have very important roles to play in the structure and function of the body. In fact essential fats may even help improve the body's metabolism and reduce the likelihood of getting fat.

So you see it is important to make sure that you and your child get enough of the right fats in the diet if they are to achieve their potential for reading, writing and learning.

Essential fats are not only important for brain function. They also play an important role in the immune system and help hormones in the body to work properly.

It can be very confusing deciding not only which fats to eat, but also how much to eat and from which foods. I will explain.

There are several different types of fat in the diet. These include saturated fats, monounsaturated fats, polyunsaturated fats and trans fats.

3.4 Saturated Fats

Saturated fats come from animal products like meat, butter, cheese, whole milk, cream and other dairy products. They also come from foods that contain these as ingredients, such as pastries, biscuits, cakes and chocolate.

It is not essential to have saturated fat in the diet. Our bodies do not need it. In fact, too much of this type of fat can pose a risk to health. It can also take the place of better, more useful essential fats.

Fats which are solid at room temperature like the saturated fats are more damaging than oils that are liquid at room temperature. Compare lard with olive oil. Lard going round your blood stream is not going to be healthy. It will be clogging your arteries and contributing to the likelihood of strokes and heart attacks.

3.5 Monounsaturated Fats

Monounsaturated fats are found in olives, olive oil, groundnut oil and avocados. Like saturated fats, they are not essential in the diet however they do not pose the same health risks if eaten in excess. In fact some studies have found they may have a beneficial effect on health if they are included in the diet, so there is no harm in using olive oil based salad dressings and adding an avocado or some olives to your salads.

3.6 Polyunsaturated Fats: essential

Polyunsaturated fats are the essential fats. They are called essential because we must get them from our diets. Our bodies can not make them.

Polyunsaturated fats mainly come from nuts, seeds and oily fish. You may have heard of Omega 3 and Omega 6 fats; these are the most well known essential polyunsaturated fats.

3.7 Omega 3

Omega 3 fats are found in fish like salmon, mackerel, sardines, herring, trout and fresh tuna.

They are also found in flax seeds.

3.8 Omega 6

Omega 6 fats are found in sunflower, sesame and pumpkin seeds or the oils of these seeds.

They are also found in almonds, walnuts, brazil and hazelnuts. The fats most beneficial to health and in particular brain health are the Omega 3 fats. Two in particular are especially important, DHA and EPA. These fats play a vital role in the physical makeup of the brain and how it functions.

The best direct sources of DHA and EPA are oily fish or fish oil supplements (not Cod Liver Oil though). Ideally you and your child should aim to eat two to three servings of oily fish a week. This could mean grilled salmon for dinner on Tuesday, mackerel on toast for breakfast on Thursday, and sardine fish cakes for lunch on Saturday. You could also eat eggs rich in Omega 3 that have come from hens fed an Omega 3 rich diet. You see, it is very easy to get essential fats into the diet.

It is best not to eat more than three servings of oily fish a week and if you are pregnant or a female planning to become pregnant in the future the advice is no more than two.

Karen says: *This is because if fish have been living in polluted sea waters they can often be contaminated with substances known as dioxins and PCBS's.*

Dioxins, PCBs and other similar chemicals are found practically everywhere, they are present in the atmosphere, soil and rivers and so easily enter the food chain. They are produced by chemical processes and come mainly from waste incinerators, chemical and fertiliser manufacturing plants.

Although in recent years the production and release of new dioxins and PCBs has reduced considerably due to an increased awareness of their dangers to human health, there is still a risk of exposure to them because they do not easily degrade or break down. Instead they remain persistent in the environment and once they get into the food chain can become stored in animal or human fat.

3.9 Omega 3

As they are fat soluble substances they are easily stored in fat. So oily fish, which contain a high level of fat, namely of the Omega 3 type, can accumulate these chemicals in their bodies. The concern with dioxin, PCB's and similar chemicals is that if they build up over time in our bodies they may have the potential to cause cancer, affect reproductive health particularly in males, may be related to behavioural problems and may increase the incidence of diabetes.

They may also affect the health of the unborn baby which is why pregnant women and females who intend to have children in the future should limit their intake of oily fish to reduce the possibility of these chemicals building up in their bodies.

Don't let this panic you and prevent you from eating oily fish though! The levels you are likely to be exposed to over a lifetime provided you stick to the recommended servings are considered safe.

The benefits of eating two to three servings of Omega 3 rich oily fish per week far outweigh the risks. However, if for some reason your child needs extra Omega 3 oils, it is best to take them in supplement form from a quality supplement manufacturer rather then eating more oily fish as any contaminants like dioxins and PCB's have been removed. Some people opt to obtain their Omega 3 fats from flax seeds. Although this bypasses the risk of potential contamination from polluted seas, the essential fats DHA and EPA may not be so easily available to the body.

3.10 Vegetarian

If your child is vegetarian flax seeds can provide some DHA and EPA, but the body must first convert the fat found in flax seeds (ALA) into DHA and EPA. Unfortunately this process may not always be sufficiently efficient and vegetarians are often low in these vital fats. Ensuring a good intake of all the other vitamins and minerals that the body needs will help towards making this conversion process go more smoothly.

Some studies have found that children with learning and behavioural problems may be less efficient at converting these fats, so supplementation, under the guidance of a nutritional therapist, with EPA and DHA directly may be necessary. Omega 6 fats have some use in the body but we do not need as much of these, in fact too many can do more harm than good.

To ensure an adequate intake I always recommend to my patients that they have either a small handful of nuts and flax seeds every day.

- Sprinkle them on breakfast or salads.
- Put them in the blender with other ingredients and make a drink.
- Snack on them.

As essential fats are easily damaged by light, heat and oxygen, it is best to keep seeds and nuts either in the refrigerator if you have room or in a dark, cool, dry place such as an airtight container in a cupboard away from any source of heat. Alternatively, you could fill a jam jar or similar glass container with the mixed ground seeds and store this in the refrigerator ready to sprinkle when you wish.

3.11 Omega 3:6 balance

Today our diets are typically overloaded with Omega 6 fats, with insufficient amounts of Omega 3. Eating a healthy, natural diet based on wholefoods, lean meat, oily fish, fruit and vegetables with very little processed, ready to eat foods will help to ensure the balance between Omega 6 and Omega 3 remains as it should. Some children however may be so deficient in the essential Omega 3 brain fats DHA and EPA that supplementation under the advice of a qualified nutritional therapist may be needed for a period of time to replenish the stores.

3.12 Benefits of essential Fats

Essential fats have many beneficial effects in the body, here are some of the key ones:

- ESSENTIAL FOR PROPER BRAIN FUNCTION. IN OTHER WORDS THEY CAN HELP WITH VISION, LEARNING ABILITY, COORDINATION, MOOD AND BEHAVIOUR.
- Improve immune function and metabolism
- Reduce the risk of allergies, asthma and eczema
- Reduce the risk of cancer, heart disease, arthritis, depression, fatigue, infections and more
- Reduce pain and inflammation
- Reduce the likelihood and severity of premenstrual symptoms by helping to balance the hormones
- Really do nurture the body, AS YOU CAN SEE.

See how important these are? So you can see, if a child is deficient, they are likely to be unwell.

And so are you. Make them a part of your routine EVERY DAY.

3.13 Trans fats

Now a bit about trans fats. These are the really bad ones and should be avoided totally. They rarely occur in natural food but if they do they are in tiny amounts and do not cause harm. However trans fats are found in large amounts in processed and deep-fried foods. They are actually monounsaturated or polyunsaturated fats that have either been damaged by high temperatures as in the case of deep frying or have been synthetically changed to make them spread easier, extend their shelf life or make them more suitable for baking.

The body is unable to make use of trans fats. They still get incorporated into the body like the good fats but they do not work in the same way. They even block the body's ability to make use of the good fats, for example they can block the conversion of ALA found in flax seeds to EPA and DHA.

Trans fats must be avoided if you want your child to be healthy and have a quick thinking and responsive brain.

Chemical messengers in the brain, the neurotransmitters, rely on brain cells having the right fats in their cell walls in order to transmit their messages. Having trans fats in the cell walls is like hitting a brick wall – the messages do not get processed.

Trans fats are generally listed on ingredient labels as hydrogenated or partially hydrogenated vegetable oils. You can also be sure that trans fats are found in most margarine, crackers and other baked goods, cookies, snack food, fast and fried foods and other processed foods. In the US and Canada the amount of trans fats in a food must now be declared on the label.

Trans fats not only provide no known benefit to human health, they actually actively contribute to poor health, raising cholesterol levels and the risk of heart disease. They have also been linked to an increased risk of cancer, Alzheimer's disease, obesity, diabetes and hormone imbalances.

A child with learning or behavioural problems certainly does not need them; they may even be contributing to his or her problems.

The only time I recommend using a saturated fat is for cooking. Ideally you would not be frying or deep frying your foods as these are not healthy ways to cook but sometimes you may need a little fat to stop food from sticking to the pan. Never use polyunsaturated fats to cook with; their delicate fats will become damaged by the high heat.

Olive oil, a monounsaturated fat, is ok to use but still can get damaged at high temperatures.

Saturated fats are not damaged by high temperatures so remain stable. I either use a little butter or I use a vegetable source saturated fat namely coconut oil.

Nutrition for Special Needs

Coconut oil has some beneficial health qualities in itself so this is my fat of choice for cooking with. I only need to use a small amount.

Neurotransmitters
4

So what about those chemical messengers in the brain, the neurotransmitters, you may well be asking now? You could be forgiven for thinking that only brain specialists should be interested in neurotransmitters but when you see what an important role they play in the brain you will understand how relevant they are in your child's learning, mood and behaviour. Brain cells communicate with each other by neurotransmitters and the overall balance of all the different types of neurotransmitters circulating in the brain at any one time affects our mood, our ability to learn, our memory, our behaviour, even our energy levels and mental alertness.

There are literally hundreds of different neurotransmitters and neurotransmitter like chemicals in the brain and some are better known than others. You may have heard of adrenalin. It's what gives us the boost we need when we have a 100m sprint to run or a crisis to deal with.

4.1 Adrenalin

But it's not just there for racing and crises. Adrenalin is a neurotransmitter and along with two other neurotransmitters, noradrenalin and dopamine, makes us feel good, motivates and stimulates us and helps us to deal with stressful situations. If there are low levels of these neurotransmitters in the brain the opposite can occur, we could feel low, even depressed, tired, apathetic and unmotivated and we may feel unable to cope with stressful situations.

If your child is feeling like this, they will most certainly not be in the mood to learn new skills such as reading or writing and may even appear lazy.

On the other hand, you wouldn't want to have too much of those stimulating neurotransmitters running about. Too much adrenalin could make your child restless, even agitated or anxious, and lacking the ability to concentrate.

4.2 GABA, serotonin, acetylcholine

Luckily the brain also has calming neurotransmitters to counteract the effects of the stimulating ones. You may have heard of GABA. This neurotransmitter has a calming and relaxing effect. A calm mind is better able to focus and concentrate. Another well known neurotransmitter is serotonin. Serotonin improves our mood and keeps us feeling happy and positive. Too little serotonin and we can feel miserable and depressed.

There is even a neurotransmitter responsible for memory, it's called acetylcholine. Too little acetylcholine in the brain and your child is very likely to be forgetful, and may even struggle to remember what he or she learnt in school.

Now you can begin to see how the balance between the different neurotransmitters can have a profound effect on how our brains work, how we think, feel and behave and also how they can affect your child's ability to learn.

4.3 Amino Acids

Neurotransmitters are mainly made from amino acids which come from the protein in our diets.

There are many sources of protein, not just meat and cheese. Eggs, lentils, beans, peas, rice, quinoa (pronounced "keenwah"), grains, yoghurt, nuts and seeds and some vegetables all contribute to the protein intake of our diets.

The most important aspect of protein is its amino acid content. Of the 23 amino acids known to exist, eight are essential. Like the essential fats, this means they must come from our diets as our bodies are unable to make them.

The amino acid content of different proteins varies and although it is extremely rare in the Western world for someone in otherwise good health to have a protein deficiency it is possible for people to be low in certain amino acids.

Different amino acids make different neurotransmitters. If your diet is continuously low or lacking in certain amino acids because you are not eating enough good quality protein on a regular basis, you may have inadequate levels of the neurotransmitters that need those amino acids to be made.

Making amino acids into neurotransmitters often takes several steps in the body and certain vitamins and minerals are needed to ensure this conversion process goes as it should. If any of those vitamins and minerals are lacking, the conversion of amino acids into neurotransmitters may be impaired and may result in a deficiency of certain neurotransmitters in the brain. The best way to ensure you and your child are getting enough of the essential amino acids in your diet and that they are being converted to neurotransmitters in the body is to eat a healthy and varied diet.

That means plenty of fruit, vegetables, seeds, nuts and a little unrefined whole grain, also by eating a serving of protein at each meal.

This could mean an egg for breakfast, tuna and kidney bean salad for lunch and a grilled chicken breast with vegetables and brown rice for dinner. Too much protein can have a negative effect on health so don't over do it thinking more will be better!

Karen says: As well as being a good source of the essential amino acids, eggs also contain good levels of a special type of fat called phospholipids.

Phospholipids help make the myelin sheath which is the fatty covering that protects and insulates nerve cells and fibres. This insulating covering ensures nerve signals and messages travel quickly and smoothly within the brain and nervous system, which makes for a quick thinking and sharp mind.

A particular kind of phospholipid, phosphatidylcholine or PC for short, still found in eggs, helps to make that all important neurotransmitter responsible for memory: acetylcholine.

So you see, eggs are positively a super brain food!

Eggs are best eaten lightly boiled, scrambled or poached to prevent the delicate fats being damaged by heat. Fried eggs I'm afraid are not a good option. It is quite safe for your child to eat up to eight eggs a week. If your child refuses to eat eggs, phospholipids are also found in sardines or can be supplemented using lecithin, available in granules from good health food stores which can be sprinkled on to food or blended into smoothies.

Many people are still wary of eating too many eggs because they contain cholesterol.

Cholesterol is needed by the body to make hormones and cell membranes and new research has now shown that cholesterol from eggs does not actually raise levels of the undesirable LDL cholesterol in the blood. (http://www.goeim.com/edelman/incredibleedibleegg_press_release/020608/index3.htm)l.

Protein
5

Having been a meat eater, a vegetarian a vegan, a vegetarian and then a chicken and some fish eater, in that order, I do have some opinions about meat. But opinions are not science. There are proven links with a diet high in red and highly processed meats and cancers of the bowel. So if you do eat meat, a little organic red meat every now and then is fine.

White meat is generally the healthier option and that means chicken and turkey, organic of course. White fish and oily fish are other good healthy sources of protein.

Although white fish like cod, plaice, hake or sea bass do not contain anywhere near as much Omega 3 fats as oily fish, white fish is a particularly good source of essential minerals like iodine and selenium as well as protein.

The healthiest way to cook fish is lightly poached, baked or grilled. Not fried and not battered. The occasional fish and chips dinner is ok, but don't forget to add some peas, tomato slices or corn on the cob to make it a healthier meal.

Fish with a breadcrumb coating might be the only way you can get your child to eat white fish, this is ok as long as you check the ingredients list and pick the ones with the most natural ingredients.

Unlike the case with oily fish there really is no limit on how much white fish to eat but there is a word of caution.

Fish that have been living in polluted sea waters can also be contaminated with low levels of the heavy metal mercury. Although mercury does occur naturally in the environment in small amounts, its levels in some waters have risen significantly over the years. Mercury is used in many chemical processes and reaches the sea either by emissions from industrial processes, the illegal dumping of industrial and chemical wastes or accidents.

Mercury is a very toxic heavy metal and has been linked with mental problems from depression, learning difficulties and loss of coordination to even madness in extremely high levels.

The level of mercury progressively increases the higher up the food chain you go. Mercury tends to be deposited at the ocean floor, small fish feed off the ocean floor and big fish eat lots of small fish. So, bigger fish that have lived (and therefore eaten) for a longer time will have accumulated higher levels of mercury in their bodies.

So the advice is not to eat too much of the big fish on a regular basis. The big fish include tuna, swordfish, shark and marlin. Children should avoid eating shark, swordfish and marlin altogether because the mercury levels in these fish could affect the development of their nervous systems.

Personally I don't know many people, let alone children who eat shark, swordfish and marlin on a regular basis but tuna is a popular fish in both the UK and US. My advice would be to limit tuna to 1 fresh tuna steak and 3 medium sized cans of tuna per month.

Karen says: Did you know that fresh tuna is classed as an oily fish whereas tinned tuna is not?

This is because the canning process reduces the Omega 3 levels of tuna. The occasional tin of tuna is ideal as a protein serving but tinned sardines, mackerel and pilchards are better sources of Omega 3. Plus being smaller fish, they will be less contaminated with mercury.

Our bodies are actually capable of dealing with a certain amount of toxic heavy metals like mercury, lead and aluminium. Having a diet that is rich in the good minerals like zinc, selenium, magnesium and calcium counterbalances the undesirable heavy metals and prevents their absorption and build up in the body.

A diet rich in vitamin C and other natural compounds found in our foods like apples, onions, garlic and eggs can also help the body to remove these unwanted metals. Fibre and water also play an important role in speeding up their removal.

Excess levels of heavy metals have been associated with mood swings, aggressive behaviour, poor attention span, impaired memory, sleep disturbance, poor impulse control and depression.

It is possible to gain an indication of the levels of toxic metals that a person has in their body by analysing a sample of hair. It is a relatively easy and cheap way of finding out if heavy metal accumulation could be a factor in your child's health.

Most nutritional therapists would be able to arrange this for you, and would then tailor a specific diet and supplement program to help speed up the removal of those heavy metals from the body.

The reasons for eating a healthy diet full of natural organic produce just keep on growing.

Vegetarians tend to opt for cheese as their source of protein but this contains too much saturated fat as well. Their best option is to ensure that throughout the course of a week they eat plenty of beans, peas, lentils, rice, quinoa and fermented soya products such as tempeh and miso.

Many ready made vegetarian foods contain trans fats or are high in saturated fats, they may also contain many other synthetic flavour enhancers or additives so they are best avoided where possible.

The best option for good health is to go for homemade vegetarian dishes. Many of which can be made in bulk and frozen ready for use when you know you will not have time to prepare and cook a meal.

Although it is possible to supplement with individual amino acids to assist the body in increasing its manufacture of certain neurotransmitters this should only be done under the guidance of a qualified nutritional therapist especially where children are concerned.

So remember, one of the best ways for most children to help keep their neurotransmitters in balance is to ensure that they are eating a healthy and varied diet, with a good source of protein at each meal.

Protein not only provides the amino acids necessary to make neurotransmitters, these amino acids are also used by the body to build, maintain and repair all of the body's tissues. It is essential therefore that a growing child gets enough protein in their diet.

There's another good reason to eat a serving of protein at each meal. It helps to keep blood sugar balanced.

It is extremely important for both physical and mental good health to keep our blood sugar balanced. I'll explain why.

As well as being used to make new tissues and substances like neurotransmitters, the food we eat is also used to produce energy.

Our bodies need energy every single second of the day just to keep functioning. We use up energy breathing, seeing, digesting, thinking and even making neurotransmitters. For our immune system to work efficiently it requires energy.

In order to create this energy our body needs a fuel, much like a car needs petrol/gas. The main source of fuel that our bodies use is called glucose.

Glucose is a type of sugar and our cells cleverly turn this sugar into usable energy so that important functions of the body can be carried out.

In order for the glucose to reach the cells it must first be absorbed from our digestive tracts into the bloodstream and carried in the blood to the various cells of the body, hence its name 'blood sugar'.

Carbohydrates and blood sugar
6

I've told you briefly about the importance of certain fats and proteins in the diet, well there is another major food group that we humans need to survive and that's carbohydrate.

Carbohydrates are the main source of sugars in our diet. There are different types of carbohydrates and some are better for you than others and I will explain why in a little while.

Keeping blood sugar balanced means there is a steady supply of glucose available to the cells to make energy. The brain in particular needs a constant supply of glucose to keep working effectively. It uses more glucose than any other organ and is not able to store it, so needs a continuous steady supply.

If our blood sugar levels drop too low it can lead to feelings of hunger, tiredness, irritability, fuzzy thinking and possibly blurred vision, not to mention poor concentration and memory. In some cases it can even lead to depression, anxiety and insomnia.

However, having high blood sugar levels is not ideal either. The body can only use a certain amount of glucose at any one time. The cells prefer to be drip fed glucose steadily so too much glucose in the blood stream does not produce more energy.

In fact what happens is the excess glucose that is not required for energy gets stored away as fat for use as a fuel in the future when food may not be so readily available.

Storing excess glucose as fat for future use as a fuel in times of food scarcity worked well for our caveman ancestors when food was often in short supply but with our modern diets being as they are, there rarely is a time of food scarcity and so these fat stores of fuel are unlikely to be used. Instead they tend to just get bigger and bring with it their own health issues.

Some studies have even linked imbalances in blood sugar levels with aggressive and hyperactive behaviour in some children.

So you see how important it is to keep your child's blood sugar balanced, especially if they are having problems with learning or concentrating at school.

Karen says: Our bodies are generally well equipped to deal with moderate rises and drops in blood sugar. The blood sugar regulating hormone insulin is responsible for keeping blood sugar levels stable. Its job is to get the glucose out of the blood and into the cells where it will be used to produce energy. Problems occur however if we over stretch or over work this mechanism. This is easily done if we regularly eat meals or items of food that are particularly high in sugar. Blood sugar levels rise very rapidly causing the body to panic and overcompensate by releasing by far too much insulin. This in turn causes blood sugar levels to rapidly drop again, often to a very low level.

This is when symptoms of low blood sugar can appear and in order to combat these, our body craves a fix of sugar to bring the level back up again. But this roller coaster of ups and downs of blood sugar is not conducive to good health, nor is it helpful for good mental health.

Being on the blood sugar 'roller coaster' can mean erratic energy levels throughout the day: drowsiness; irritability and mood swings; headaches; poor concentration and memory. It also leads to cravings for sweet foods and the need for frequent meals or snacks. And so the vicious circle continues.

So what is the best way to keep you and your child's blood sugar balanced?

Earlier I said there are different types of carbohydrate, some being better for you than others.

The type of carbohydrate your child eats can have a profound effect not only on his or her energy levels but also their mental health too.

6.1 Simple/complex

The easiest way to look at carbohydrates is they are either "simple" or "complex". Simple carbohydrates break down very easily and quickly into sugar causing a more rapid increase in blood sugar levels. A correspondingly rapid drop in blood sugar levels would then ultimately follow.

Complex carbohydrates however are broken down by the body much more slowly and so give a more steady release of sugar for energy throughout the day.

Eating complex carbohydrates rather than simple carbohydrates helps you and your child to avoid that blood sugar 'roller coaster' and all the problems that come with it.

Simple carbohydrates are things like white bread, white pasta and white rice. These are refined, highly processed carbohydrates and very quickly get broken down into sugar in the body.

I probably don't need to tell you that sugar itself and foods containing sugar are a real no-no if you want to balance your body's blood sugar levels.

Sweet foods like cakes, biscuits, most breakfast cereals and cereal bars, fizzy drinks, flavoured and sweetened yoghurts, chocolate, sweets and snacks also release their sugars into the blood stream very rapidly.

In fact most processed foods contain a large amount of sugar that can wreak havoc with our blood sugar levels.

These foods should be avoided where at all possible.

Some natural foods also contain high amounts of natural sugars and ideally these should be eaten only occasionally. For example, honey, raisins, parsnips, fruit juices, bananas and melons.

The good thing about these foods though is that they also contain other nutrients that are good for us, unlike the processed refined carbohydrates.

Many people have cereals for breakfast. They are easy and the adverts tell us they are full of nutrients. In one experiment with rats, rats ate the box and left the cereal.

There is not much nutrition left in those grains when they have undergone the processing it takes to produce some of those cereals. Think about a raw piece of corn or a wheat ear, and think of some of those cereals and there is no resemblance between the two. They will not make you healthy.

Karen says: Cereal crops are 'dehulled' and processed to make breakfast cereals and bread.

This strips them of essential vitamins and minerals such as B vitamins, chromium, zinc and manganese to name but a few. The food manufacturers then add synthetic forms of the vitamins and minerals back in to make up for it.

Complex carbohydrates on the other hand are good for us. They provide a steady supply of fuel for energy as they take longer to be broken down by the body, so our blood sugar levels do not "spike" in the same way as when we eat simple carbohydrates.

They also contain more of the original nutrients of the plant. Complex carbohydrates are things like whole grains instead of refined grains so that means brown or whole grain bread, brown rice and brown pastas. Complex carbohydrates are also found in most natural unrefined plant foods like vegetables, beans and pulses. Whole grains are not "dehulled" so still contain their essential vitamins and minerals.

So eat complex carbohydrates instead of simple carbohydrates to keep blood sugar levels steady.

And avoid foods that have had sugar added to them. Beware though, sugar comes in many disguises. Always read the label and if any of the following are listed in the ingredients, then sugar has been added:

Glucose,
glucosefructose,
high fructose corn syrup,
corn syrup,
syrup,
dextrose,
dextrin,
fructose,
galactose,
maltose,
maltodextrin,
evaporated cane juice,

concentrated fruit juice,
maple syrup,
honey,
molasses,
raw cane sugar,
sucrose.
I was walking up and down the drink aisle at a supermarket yesterday trying to find lemonade that did not contain things that could potentially harm us. Every single one I looked at contained artificial sweeteners, such as aspartame or acesulfame K, or preservatives such as sodium benzoate. As I state later on, we do not eat any ingredients that were not invented by the 1940s, and these artificial ingredients were not.

Karen says: Artificial sweeteners are nothing but synthetic chemicals. Not only that, but using artificial sweeteners such as aspartame, saccharin, sucralose or acesulfame K do not help your child to reduce their craving for sweetness. It is far better to slowly wean your child off sugar by gradually using less of it than simply substituting it with synthetically made substances which are a totally alien "food" and could potentially pose a risk to health.

I mentioned earlier that protein can help keep blood sugar levels balanced too. By combining complex carbohydrates with protein at a meal the release of sugar into the blood stream is slowed down even further giving even more sustained energy. The aim of my information is to keep you healthy, and these days that means balancing blood sugar levels so that you don't crave sugar and end up eating loads of sugary foods which are usually accompanied by fat, and very little in the way of essential nutrients. I know this because I have had issues with my own blood sugar balance for years. My eating is under control now because I have found out how to do this. Eating regularly is really important. I always make sure I eat breakfast, lunch and dinner. I also have a small snack in between to keep my blood sugar on an even keel. So actually every two hours I have something to eat.

When I used to skip meals or snacks I would get hungry, a little lightheaded, unable to think so clearly, shaky, and feel a bit sleepy. So I used to grab the quickest and easiest food I could find to boost my energy.

This usually meant a chocolate or cereal bar, or a slice of white toasted bread with jam but these are high in sugar, so my blood sugar would shoot up only to tumble back down again half an hour later and the hunger, lightheadedness and shakes would soon return.

Regular eating, complex instead of simple carbohydrates with a little protein at each meal and snack keeps me feeling stable both physically and mentally. If I leave eating for more than two hours I get shaky and irritable.

Your child may be experiencing these same symptoms too.

This is why they may throw irritable tantrums at certain times of the day and can only be placated by a chocolate bar or other similar candy.

It might be why they lose concentration and the ability to focus in class. Studies have found that children who eat a healthy breakfast have better attention spans and concentration levels than those that do not.

A hearty breakfast provides your child with the necessary fuel to function effectively throughout the morning. It ensures the brain is supplied with a steady supply of glucose to keep thinking clear and focused.

6.1 Sleep, energy

Remember, unbalanced blood sugar levels means erratic energy and concentration levels. They can also disrupt healthy sleeping patterns. It goes without saying that a child who has had a good night's sleep stands a much better chance of being able to concentrate and focus at school than a child whose sleep has been interrupted.

Feeling sleepy during the day, awake and bounding with energy late at night or waking during the night but sleepy again when it's time to get up can all be indications that blood sugar levels are out of control.

A child needs on average nine to 12 hours, depending on their age, of good quality sleep a night.

Nutrition for Special Needs

Without sufficient sleep a child's immune system can be weakened making them more prone to infections and illnesses. As well as reducing their ability to concentrate and think clearly they can also become irritable and moody. Sleep is vital for growing children. Without adequate sleep physical growth and mental development can be impaired.

Drinks
7

Don't forget about drinks either.

These too can upset blood sugar balance.

Water is preferred. Clean water with nothing added and not in a plastic bottle. Plastic can leach dioxins and Bisphenol A into the water. These are not healthy.

Nowadays, water sold in the shops can come with all sorts of flavours added, and often sweeteners are added too so beware.

Water is a crucial factor in good health. All the chemical reactions that take place every day at every level in the body are governed by enzymes and these enzymes need water to work properly. Water keeps every cell, tissue and organ in the body moist, flexible and healthy. It also helps the body to flush out toxins and other unwanted waste and so has a beneficial cleansing effect.

Tuning in to our body's needs when we are used to tuning it out can take some getting used to.

If you or your child have been used to having sugary drinks that give instant energy, then getting used to plain water might take a while. Fruit juices come second to water. The ones you make yourself, fresh, are best. Most readymade juices sold in cartons are pasteurised to kill germs, and the pasteurisation also kills enzymes.

Karen says: These enzymes are what make food alive and good for us. The enzymes from fruits and vegetables support the function of our own enzymes. Also the fresh home made juice will contain more vitamins and minerals. The pasteurisation process may also destroy these.

Fruits naturally contain sugar, and commercial fruit juices generally contain high amounts. The processing of the fruit to make the juice concentrates the sugar. If you are trying to reduce your child's sugar intake, then dilute fruit juices with water, or use a smaller glass.

But remember, eating the whole fruit is always much better for you than just extracting and drinking its juice. The whole fruit contains fibre and other beneficial nutrients which are lost when you only drink the juice.

So give your child water to drink whenever possible.

If you must add something to their water, add a good organic squash. Be warned though that some children react with oranges and lemons, so the blackcurrant ones might be better. I will talk more later about allergies and intolerances.

Those are the good things a child should drink. Water and homemade juice. Sometimes we put some organic squash with hot water for a warming winter drink too.

7.1 Stimulants

I really would suggest that you don't give drinks with sugar or caffeine to your children. Caffeine is a stimulant and has a similar effect on blood sugar levels as sugar. Why does a child need stimulants? They do not.

Caffeine is not just found in coffee. It's also found in tea and many canned drinks like cola so always read the label.

Chocolate is made from cocoa which contains some caffeine as well as another stimulant, theobromine. Theobromine is also found in coffee. Decaff versions are actually not much better as they still contain some caffeine, just less than regular versions and the other stimulants are still kept in.

The South African Redbush or Rooibos tea is a good stimulant free alternative to regular tea. It also doesn't contain tannins which regular tea does. Tannins are chemical compounds found in many plants but they can, if eaten or drunk in large quantities, interfere with the absorption of essential minerals in the digestive system. I expect you are wondering why I have not included cow's milk for that all important calcium.

7.2 Milk

Breast milk is of course the best food for a newborn baby but I look at it like this: if a person is weaned they do not need milk. They especially do not need milk from another species that turns a large baby calf into a huge animal in eighteen months.

Cow's milk is designed for baby cows not baby humans. It is far too rich and full of compounds that promote rapid growth in baby calves and therefore really not suitable for human children.

Cow's milk is often found to cause allergies, intolerances or digestive problems. It has also been linked to other common childhood ailments such as eczema, asthma and glue ear.

Some people have problems digesting lactose, the sugar in cow's milk. Others are unable to handle the milk protein, casein. I will talk more about these allergies and intolerances a little later but my belief is that, reducing or even avoiding cow's milk is the safest option.

But what about the calcium you still ask?

7.3 Magnesium, calcium

Karen says: Milk may have a high calcium content but for calcium to be effectively used by the body it needs to be in the right balance with magnesium. Milk has very little magnesium. Magnesium deficiency is extremely common in children. Otherwise known as the relaxing mineral, magnesium helps maintain healthy muscles, it is also vital for energy production, nerve function and mental health.

Magnesium deficiency signs include muscle weakness, insomnia, nervousness and constipation.

Dark green leafy vegetables which contain magnesium, not to mention other minerals as well, are a much better source of calcium. Sardines, salmon, broccoli, beans, seeds and nuts are also all good sources of calcium.

Another reason why milk is promoted as good for children is its high calorie content and because it's viewed as a complete food – containing protein, carbohydrate and fat.

However it does lack many other important nutrients and filling up on milk each day could prevent your child from eating a more varied and nutritious diet. Everything that milk provides plus more can be obtained from other foods.

7.4 Nut and seed milks

So you see, there really is little reason to drink cow's milk, especially if you are eating a healthy and varied diet.

There are times when a 'milk' is needed and there are alternatives. We use rice milk in our porridge.

If you have a blender, nut milks make a very tasty nourishing drink. Obviously if you have a nut allergy avoid this.

In the blender I put a glass of water and a handful of sesame, sunflower, flax and pumpkin seeds as a base. Then add any other nuts I feel like adding that day. Blend till smooth. Yum, yum.

You can buy readymade nut milks, rice milk or oat milk from the health food store.

7.5 Soya

Soya milk is often suggested as an alternative to cow's milk but I believe the jury is still out on soya, especially the soya milk and soya products that are available in our supermarkets in the West. There is a lot of controversy and confusion about soya and it's effects on human health.

Many of the reports on the benefits of consuming soya are based upon observations in Eastern populations such as the Japanese and Chinese that have a long tradition of eating soy based foods and a low incidence of certain cancers and other health issues. In addition the lack of reported adverse effects from eating soy in these populations has prompted many in the West to assume that soy is safe.

An important but often neglected distinction between soy products consumed in the West and those eaten traditionally in the East is that the soya is eaten in its fermented form in the East, and in small amounts. In the West however, soya is not fermented and is eaten in much larger quantities by many people, either as a replacement protein for meat and dairy or through its addition to a multitude of processed foods.

The soya products available to us today in the West are quite likely to have originated from genetically modified soya crops and are highly refined and processed. Like anything that has been refined or processed, I wouldn't eat or drink too much of it.

Vitamins and Minerals
8

So I've told you all about the major nutrients fat, protein and carbohydrate and their importance to your child's health and mental well being. But what about all the smaller nutrients like vitamins and minerals and other substances found in our food that may or may not be beneficial to us?

Many of these smaller nutrients are just as important to good health as the big ones. Remember vitamins and minerals are needed by the body on a daily basis to help make those important brain chemicals, the neurotransmitters.

They're also needed to enable the body to make use of the essential fats and some like chromium and magnesium are even needed to help keep blood sugar levels balanced.

Without an adequate supply of vitamins and minerals our bodies struggle to turn the food we eat into energy for physical and mental activity.

Vitamins and minerals also perform some less obvious but nonetheless important functions in the body, and there are quite possibly other functions of vitamins and minerals that we haven't discovered yet.

Vitamin A

Vitamin A for example is essential for healthy skin and a strong immune system, but it is also crucial for proper vision and healthy eyes. Ensuring good eyesight is important when dealing with children with learning or coordination difficulties. Vitamin A also contributes to the health of the lining of the digestive tract which can influence your child's risk of developing allergies or intolerances and can also have an impact on your child's mental health. I will explain more about this a little later.

Vitamin D

Vitamin D is an interesting one. Scientists now consider it to be a hormone rather than a vitamin because of the extent to which it works in the body. Until a few years ago, most people thought Vitamin D was only essential to prevent the bone disease rickets, but a group of scientists in the U.S. looking at the benefits of vitamin D for brain health discovered that Vitamin D has an important role in the development and function of the brain.

They found that vitamin D can affect certain proteins in the brain involved in learning, memory, muscle control and even behaviour. Although it is still not clear exactly how vitamin D works in the brain, the presence of a large number of vitamin D receptors in the brain implies that it may indeed have an important role in maintaining brain health.

Technically we should get most of our vitamin D from the sun rather than the diet. The skin is able to manufacture vitamin D when it is exposed to sufficient sunlight. However, especially in northern latitudes such as in the UK and Northern Europe, we do not get enough sunshine. On top of that with the increased fear of getting skin cancer, we now cover our skin up with clothes and sun screens to further lessen our exposure to the sun.

Some scientists are now looking to see whether or not there is a link between the mother's exposure to sun and hence vitamin D levels and behavioural problems in their children.

Magnesium

Some of the symptoms of magnesium deficiency bear a striking resemblance to some of the symptoms seen in children with ADHD. Although magnesium may not be the whole answer to the problem, it could be that inadequate levels of magnesium could be making the situation worse. Restlessness, anxiety, insomnia, fidgeting, muscle twitches, coordination problems and learning difficulties are all symptoms of magnesium deficiency.

Nutrition for Special Needs

Magnesium is known as the muscle relaxant mineral and some studies have found that it may be helpful in preventing or even treating asthma attacks as it can help to relax the muscles of the lungs.

This is just a snapshot of three nutrients. Imagine how many more pages I could write if I went into detail on all the other vitamins and minerals we need.

Our diets today
9

If your diet until now has not been one based around plenty of organic whole foods, fruit and vegetables, then you are quite possibly deficient in certain vitamins and minerals as a family, and all of you will probably benefit from following the brainbuzzz programme (www.brainbuzzz.co.uk) . Not just your hyperactive/dyspraxic/dyslexic child.

If we compare the amount of nutrients in our food now (even organically grown) with the same food grown during the Second World War, today's food is severely mineral and vitamin deficient.

In other words we can eat the same as our parents and grandparents did, and we can never be as healthy. That is one more reason why more sustainable methods of agriculture are becoming more fashionable again.

Karen says: Intensive farming has destroyed our soils and depleted their nutrient content by the indiscriminate use of chemicals and poor soil management.

We get our minerals from the plants and animals that we eat. The plants get the minerals from the soil in which they are grown and the animals get the minerals from the plants they eat and pass them on to us.

A fertile healthy soil is needed to produce wholesome, nutrient rich food. Modern fertilisers increase the growth and yield of crops but not their nutritious value. They only add the minerals that help plants grow taller and quicker, not the minerals that we humans actually need. To add those as well would be too costly.

The mineral selenium is particularly depleted in our soils which is a major concern because this mineral plays a key role in the body in the prevention of cancer and is vital for a healthy immune system.

It will take years to remineralise even organic soils, but it is a start. So in the meantime we need to make sure that our diets are the best they can be. One of the things we hear a lot is 'everything in moderation'. Well, I don't know about you but I don't think that makes any sense, especially as the people who quote it to me have all been alcoholics.

Moderate what? Lard? I haven't had my moderate amount of lard today that's for sure. Have you?

If we want to ensure we are getting all the nutrients our bodies need to maintain optimum health, surely a moderate amount of fruit and vegetables is not enough in this day and age? So forget that, and focus on more practical and enjoyable aspects to food.

Fundamental to our health are fresh produce grown in season and local. If it is local, then it is likelier to be more nutritious; it won't have lost its goodness on a plane from the other side of the world.

If it is in season then it is likely to be local too, and fresher. If you shop at your local farm shop it is better for all.

The diet in the Second World War was a healthy one for various reasons:

- The diet was much more basic and consisted of vegetables with a little meat and some fruit.
- It was mostly locally grown therefore it was seasonal and fresher.
- There were far less chemical fertilisers, pesticides and herbicides around. They hadn't been invented.
- It was rationed, so obesity was extremely rare.
- There was hardly any sugar and sweets were rationed

There were no harmful or chemical additives such as

- toxic colourings
- flavourings
- preservatives
- flavour enhancers
- artificial sweeteners
- thickeners

Nutrition for Special Needs

Although fresh fruit was hard to come by, and eggs were scarce, the overall diet is considered to be much healthier than today's average diet.

We have a largely Second World War diet in our house. I cook everything from fresh every day and we do not use any ingredients that were not invented since the 1940s.

We do have some international ingredients such as soy sauce, though, and that was definitely nvented before the forties.

We grow some of our own vegetables and fruit and we keep chickens. This is not possible of everyone, and certainly 'digging for victory' is hard work. But it is something I believe in. Its also great exercise.

If you have a big enough garden or an allotment, it is possible to find the actual Digging for Victory planting schedules on the internet. This method produces food for every week of the year. Amazing.

If you seek out your local farm shop or fresh fruit and vegetable shop, it is the next best thing.

This kind of shopping and production cuts down on packaging and waste AND you will be eating seasonal food too.

As soon as food is dug from the ground or picked from the plants or trees its nutrient value begins to decrease. By the time it has been packaged, transported, stored and sold in the supermarket its nutrient value is considerably lower. Add to that the storage time in your refrigerator before you eat it and the nutrient value of your vegetables is unlikely to be what you would like it to be.

Karen says: On top of that, vitamins and minerals are quite delicate molecules and are easily destroyed by heat, light and exposure to oxygen. So the best way to cook vegetables and preserve their nutrients is to lightly steam or quickly stir fry them. Some vitamins and minerals leach out into the water when food is boiled so if you do boil your vegetables, use the cooking water as the liquid for soups or casseroles.

Frozen vegetables are however one of the few 'processed/ ready made' foods that are ok to eat.

The vegetables are frozen very soon after picking and therefore their nutrients are retained.

Remember to steam rather than boil them when cooking them.

What we eat is really, really important. What we eat becomes us. The food becomes our body. If we are eating nutrient free food, then health will disappear.

What we eat is really, really important. What we eat becomes us. The food becomes our body. If we are eating nutrient free food, then health will disappear.

That is so important I have said it twice.

Now, reading about something being bad, and believing it is not the same thing. My advice is check ingredients lists on everything before you buy it.

Do not be persuaded by peer pressure.

Do not give in to people who say 'just a little bit won't hurt'

Do not give in to people who say 'just this once won't hurt'.

YES IT WILL

YES IT WILL

YES IT WILL.

Don't risk it, it is not worth it. Even check the toothpaste. Check everything. Laziness and nonchalance does not lead to good health.

I think this is really crucial and I want you to think that too. Don't keep eating the burgers and saying 'nothing wrong with this, it's just bread and meat and a bit of salad'. There is a lot wrong with that.

The white roll is so highly processed and refined (basically it's a simple carbohydrate!) it's tantamount to eating sugar. The meat most likely comes from cattle intensively reared on soya crops and fattened up with any number of synthetic substances or additives so that more burgers can be made from the one cow, and so provides more saturated fat than essential nutrients. The tiny amount of salad that has been transported, stored and refrigerated, for who knows how long, is barely enough to meet 1 serving of your recommended five fruit and vegetables servings per day.

Sourcing foods and preparing meals
10

If you are growing your own food or buying it from your local farm shop, then you are avoiding/bypassing all of the processing that takes the nutrients out of food.

When I cook from scratch I never use ingredients with long chemical names that I can't pronounce, I never need thickeners or stabilizers or acidity regulators.

They are used in foods that are readymade and will sit about for a few days. Some additives are only used to extend the shelf life of products. This means they can be made at a factory weeks before, then transported to your supermarket's warehouse, put on the shelf and still have a few days left before the ingredients start going off. During this time the food loses what little nutrients it had in the first place.

You can probably see by now that if you buy ready made foods and do not eat many fresh vegetables, then you are probably not in the optimum health you could possibly achieve. Your child could be the same.

I find that making one small change every day for a few weeks, builds up into a lot of difference over time. Before you know it, the changes will be habit.

You are probably thinking that it takes ages to cook properly. Well, I work full time, have two children and a house to run (and we won't mention the garden). I am busy, and generally don't stay on top of it all.

One week there's piles of washing and another I'm behind with the washing up. The windows don't get done often enough, and I have about ten minutes to prepare each meal.

It takes less than that to make a casserole and put it in the oven to cook. Pavlova from my own chickens' eggs takes ten minutes not including cooking. I add homegrown raspberries. Things in the oven can be ignored until the buzzer goes. Jacket potatoes take just a minute to prepare. Nothing I prepare takes more than a few minutes because I don't have the time, and yet it is all fresh and barring a few disasters; yummy.

If you follow the 'grow your own/farm shop' idea then you will be avoiding many of the problems that could come your way with poor food choices.

The simple rule is to mostly eat natural, unadulterated, local and if possible, organic, food.

10.1 Five a day

Eat plenty of vegetables and some fruit. Ideally you should eat more vegetables than fruit because fruit does naturally contain sugar. If you follow the five-day plan, it's better to eat three vegetable servings and two fruit servings per day.

Personally I don't think five-day is enough. It's a start definitely, but we should really be aiming or 10 if not 12 a day if you and your child want to achieve optimum health. That would mean seven or eight servings of vegetables and three or four servings of fruit a day.

And what constitutes a serving? Generally speaking one serving is 80g of a particular food.

Potatoes and yams do not count towards one of your fruit and vegetable servings though, they are classed as a carbohydrate a bit like rice or bread and do not offer the same level of nutrients as found in other vegetables.

Here are a few examples of one serving:

one large carrot;

one large bell pepper;

one medium sized tomato;

80g of Brussels sprouts, cabbage or broccoli;

two sticks of celery;

one apple;
two plums;
10 strawberries;
25 raspberries
or 48 blueberries.
Yes, 48 blueberries provide just one serving of your five-a-day.
How many of you eat just five to 10 blueberries and think that's
good enough?
At first this might seem impossible but you will be surprised
how easy it is to add those extra servings of vegetables and
fruit to your daily meals. Make every meal as colourful as you
can with as wide a variety of fruit and vegetables each day as
possible.
Make big salads with everything added, from the basic salad
leaves, cucumber and tomatoes to beetroot, grated carrot,
celery, red onion, avocado and a few raw broccoli florets.
Casseroles are extremely quick and easy to make. Chop all the
ingredients up, put them in a dish, add some water and herbs,
put in the oven and forget about it until the buzzer goes. Leeks,
onions, carrots, mushrooms, courgettes, squash, green beans,
tomatoes, celery are just some of the ingredients you could
use.
If your child is reluctant to eat such a wide variety of vegetables
there are ways of getting them into the diet without them being
aware. Homemade soups are easy to make, and once blended
your child will not have a clue what vegetables you've added in.
You may need to experiment with quantities of various
vegetables to get a taste your child likes though. Roasted
sweet potato and red pepper soup is always a firm favourite in
our house. But I also add onion, celery, leek and a few green
beans for good measure too. A little chilli powder or
fresh garlic can add a little excitement to the flavour.
You can add finely chopped vegetables to spaghetti bolognaise
or other pasta sauces and also to homemade
burger recipes. Most children like vegetable or fruit kebabs. Be
imaginative, creative and experimental, food can and should be
fun. Not like pushing the jelly up a hill as I said
earlier.

It often also helps if you get your children involved in the preparation and cooking process as well. It's also vitally important that our next generation actually knows how to cook home made food. My youngest is really proud of his cooking skills, and often asks to prepare a dish. He doesn't get it from me, I hated cooking as a child, but I have to do it now.

Gut health
11

Karen says: Increasing the amount of fruit and vegetables in your diet not only increases the quantity and variety of nutrients you and your child receives but also supports a healthy digestive system as they are a rich source of fibre.

Many people underestimate the importance of a healthy digestive system. The digestive tract is a barrier between the body and the outside world, much like the skin, and ensuring it remains healthy is vital in maintaining a healthy immune system and reducing the risk of allergies and food intolerances. We not only obtain vital nutrients via our digestive tracts but at the other end, we also eliminate unwanted substances.

These substances can be toxic byproducts that the body no longer wants or needs. If we don' have enough fibre in our diet, these toxins can hang around in the gut longer than they should and may even be reabsorbed
leading to a toxic buildup in the body.

11.1 Toxins, mood, fibre, probiotics

Unfortunately our delicate brains are very sensitive to toxins in the body and signs such as lethargy, mental fogginess, confusion, poor memory and low mood may be an indication that our bodies are not dealing properly with toxins.

This is why nutritional therapists are often very interested in people's poo!

Fibre not only ensures we get rid of unwanted substances on a regular basis but it also helps support the friendly bacteria that live in our digestive tracts.

There has been a lot of interest recently in the friendly bacteria of our guts and there is just cause for this.

These little critters play such an important role in our immune system that scientists have found that illnesses from cystitis to hay fever may be due to insufficient friendly bacteria in the gut. A good strong immune system will help a person remain well even when there are many opportunities to be ill. A child with a strong and healthy immune system will not be prone to every bug and infection that is going around. Their vitality and robustness will see them through while other children will have one illness after the other.

11.2 Immunity

Scientists have only just recently discovered that at least 70% or our immunity lies in the gut. On top of that, connections are now being made between the health of the gut and many other illnesses, from food intolerances, allergies, autoimmune diseases and even some behavioural and mental health issues. Imagine the digestive tract as being like a tube through which food gets passed. As it travels through it is the job of our digestive system to absorb vital nutrients from the food to keep us alive.

To enable these tiny molecules to be absorbed, the lining of the digestive 'tube' has be to quite thin and permeable. A little like a sieve, it is designed to only let very tiny molecules through, and it is therefore extremely delicate.

Unfortunately we tend to ignore this fact and regularly bombard our digestive tracts with all manner of substances. Not just natural food but also countless amounts of chemical additives that are now added to our foods, pesticide and herbicide residues present on our food, a variety of medicines, from painkillers to antibiotics, and in the case of many adults, alcohol on a regular basis too.

These substances can in many cases irritate and even damage the delicate linings our digestive tracts. They can also severely disrupt the balance of the friendly bacteria that live along the lining of our guts.

The gut lining acts as a barrier, letting good nutrients in and preventing unwanted substances from entering. If this lining is damaged in anyway, there is the increased risk that unwanted substances can get through. Don't forget also that certain nutrients are needed in the diet to maintain a healthy gut. If the diet is lacking in these nutrients in the first place there is a weakness already.

The friendly bacteria are not just there because they have nowhere else to live. They have a job to do. They produce substances that nourish and protect the cells of the digestive lining and so keep it healthy.

They produce substances that help keep levels of harmful bacteria, viruses, yeast and parasites that can also live in our digestive tracts in check. They produce B vitamins and help in the absorption of minerals. They can even eliminate substances that are potential carcinogens. They also generally help with the digestive process.

Karen says: Chewing food, the digestive juices such as saliva and stomach acid and those released into the stomach and small intestines, together with muscular contractions of the digestive tract all help to break down our food into very tiny molecules.

If we don't chew our food sufficiently, which is often the case nowadays as far too many of us eat in a rush, gulping our food down as soon as it's put into the mouth, the first stage of digestion does not take place. Who ever heard of stomachs having teeth?

Children are also likely to not chew their food properly. Either they are not aware of the need to chew their food to the point of it being almost liquid in their mouths (I like to think of it as 'at least 15 chomps of the teeth' should be sufficient) or they too are in a hurry to go off and do something more interesting instead or they may simply just be distracted from the process of eating by the TV.

Improperly digested food can in itself irritate the delicate lining of the digestive tract. Undigested food can also become a source of food for the more 'unfriendly' types of bacteria that also reside in our guts. If the delicate balance between our 'friendly' and 'unfriendly' bacteria is tipped in the wrong direction, this could mean the unfriendly bacteria could multiply quite rapidly and health problems will develop.

So you can see there are already some very good reasons why it is important to keep you and your child's digestive system in good order.

11.3 Intolerances, allergies, mental function

But how does this all link up with allergies, food intolerances and mental function you might be asking?

There are a number of factors that may be involved.

An irritated, inflamed or damaged gut lining will not be well equipped to properly absorb the essential nutrients our bodies need to keep healthy. Deficiencies in certain nutrients can cause the immune system not to work as it should not to mention all the other functions our bodies perform.

If the lining of the gut is not as healthy as it should be and substances that would not normally get through do, these could trigger a reaction from the immune system as it will not recognise them and sees them as foreign invaders.

In most cases, food allergies and sensitivities develop as a result of the immune system reacting to certain protein molecules found in food. Protein molecules are found in many foods, not just the main protein foods.

Generally proteins get broken down by a healthy digestive system into amino acids and it is these tiny amino acid molecules that are normally allowed to pass through our gut linings and into the bloodstream. Our immune systems recognise these small amino acids as 'friends' rather than 'foes' and so do not react.

If the lining is damaged, some of the larger unbroken protein molecules from our foods get through and pass into the blood stream triggering reactions from the immune system.

These protein molecules once in the blood stream can interact with other parts of the body too and in particular the brain.

There has been some interest in the proteins in gluten found in grains and casein found in milk which if not properly digested can turn into substances which have a very similar chemical structure to opiates like morphine or heroin.

These substances can pass through the blood brain barrier and disrupt the normal functioning of the brain. Some studies have detected the presence of these substances in the urine of people with schizophrenia, autism, ADHD, depression and Down's syndrome.

It is important to remember however that everyone is unique and that many different factors combined can contribute to a person's physical and mental well being but ensuring your child's digestive system is as healthy as it can be seems a good place to start.

The difference between food allergy and food intolerance is generally the type and level of reaction.

A true food allergy results in a severe and immediate reaction, it may even be life-threatening.

Often these kinds of allergies are lifelong and the offending food must be avoided at all times. If your child has such an allergy I am sure you are already well aware of it.

This type of allergy may not necessarily be as a result of an unhealthy digestive system but keeping the digestive tract healthy may prevent the risk of further allergies or intolerances developing. It will also help keep the immune system otherwise healthy and support overall health as well.

Another type of allergy results in less severe and less immediate symptoms. They could even develop over the course of several days; this makes it very difficult to determine the culprit.

Generally these types of reaction are known as delayed onset. Symptoms are usually quite minor and may even go undetected. These are the allergies most commonly associated with problems in the digestive tract and improving the health of the digestive system can make a considerable difference.

Food intolerances or sensitivities generally do not elicit a direct response from the immune system although they can still produce uncomfortable or undesirable symptoms.

11.4 Lactose intolerance

For example lactose intolerance; some people are unable to properly digest lactose the sugar found in milk as they lack the enzyme needed to digest it.

Symptoms such as bloating, abdominal discomfort and diarrhoea may occur. Again improving the health and supporting the digestive system and making changes to the diet can result in reduced symptoms.

If you suspect your child may have a food allergy or intolerance it may be a good idea to keep a food and symptom diary for a few weeks, writing down the foods eaten and any symptoms or behavioural changes that you notice.

There are some common culprits though. These are wheat and other gluten grains, milk and milk products, both of which I will tell you more about in a little while, also eggs, foods containing yeast, shellfish, citrus fruits, chocolate, nuts, peanuts and soya. Certain food additives have also been known to result in sensitivity reactions.

It is estimated that almost one in three children with behavioural problems have food allergies or sensitivities. It can be quite difficult to determine which food or foods are causing the reactions so if you suspect food allergy or intolerances could be contributing to your child's poor health or behavioural problems I would recommend that you see a nutritional therapist for more detailed advice.

Problem Foods
12

12.1 Gluten

There are some foods however that I believe if eaten on a daily basis are detrimental to the health of everyone. The first one is wheat and other gluten containing grains.

Wheat and the products made from wheat although strictly classed as carbohydrate, contain a protein complex called gluten.

Gluten is a sticky, hard to digest substance that can place a real strain on the digestive systems of most humans. Gluten is also found in rye, barley, oats and spelt.

Some people have a true allergy to gluten and can become quite ill if they do not avoid gluten altogether. These people have what is called coeliac disease where gluten causes severe damage to the intestinal lining.

This interferes with the absorption of essential nutrients to such a degree that those suffering from the condition, if undiagnosed and still eating gluten, will loose weight and or already be very thin, suffer from severe fatigue, depression, mental fogginess, diarrhoea or constipation and intestinal gas, bloating and discomfort not to mention many other possible symptoms.

Anyone with suspected coeliac disease should seek professional medical and nutritional advice.

There are however increasing numbers of adults and children who although they do not have coeliac disease do find they are sensitive to the gluey protein and find that many of their physical and mental problems improve when they significantly reduce the amount of gluten and wheat they eat.

Nutrition for Special Needs

Gluten is found in many foods not just wheat and cereal based products. It's used as a stabilising agent in products like ice-cream and ketchup and can be found in many processed foods.

There is another reason why I don't like wheat. Our diet has become very dependent on wheat and cereal based grains over the last 10,000 years even though genetically we are still 'huntergatherers'.

Huntergatherers did not eat cereal grains, as agriculture had not been invented back then.

Nowadays we eat wheat or cereal based foods at every opportunity. For breakfast we eat cereals, for snacks we eat biscuits made with wheat, for lunches we have sandwiches and at dinner we have wheat pasta or pizza bases. Not to mention the many other foods that wheat or wheat flour gets added to.

It is not good to eat too much of the same thing. The body is designed to eat a wide variety of nutrient rich foods. Wheat and cereal grains contain some nutrients although they do not contain enough or the variety to meet our needs.

By eating wheat based foods at every meal this means we are not eating other foods that we should be eating. Instead of a tuna wheat sandwich, we could be eating a tuna salad which would contain far more nutrients than the bread sandwich.

Another disadvantage with cereal grains such as wheat, is that they contain phytates. These are plant compounds that prevent the absorption of minerals such calcium and iron. So if your child's diet is already low in mineral rich foods, eating a lot of cereal based foods like bread and pasta will not be helping.

Cereals contain a large number of other plant compounds which scientists are beginning to look at and some have been shown to have detrimental effects to the health, the most well known of these is lectins.

Lectins are proteins and unlike some of the other proteins already mentioned, they can bind to cells in the body and interfere with the normal function of those cells. For example they can bind to red blood cells and cause them to clump together. A particular lectin found in wheat, wheat germ agglutinin (WGA) has been found to bind with cells in the mouth, stomach, intestines, skin, nervous system and other organs of the body.

It has been proposed that lectins could bind to cells lining the intestinal tract and therefore cause irritation and damage, which in turn may allow other protein molecules to pass through the lining and react with the body's immune system and brain. Personally I try to avoid eating too much wheat and other cereal grains where possible. Every now and then is fine, but not everyday and certainly not at every meal. Instead I eat lots more vegetables, seeds, nuts, brown rice, lentils and berries. For further reading on the effect of gluten on the brain (an inflammatory) my favourite source is the work of Loren Cordain.

12.2 Dairy products

The second food which I believe if consumed on a regular basis is detrimental to health is cows' milk. I have already explained why I don't think humans need to drink cows' milk but the fact that it is also a common cause of allergies is another good reason. Again, there are some people who have a true allergy to cows' milk and will need to avoid it and anything made from it completely. The allergy is in fact to one of the proteins found in the milk.

Others may just have lactose intolerance which means they can no longer digest or tolerate the milk sugar lactose and so suffer symptoms as a result.

Lactose intolerance is more common in adults and people from certain ethnic communities. Milk from goats and sheep also contain lactose so these are not suitable alternatives.

Some people with lactose intolerance can eat cheese and yoghurt without too many problems though. Cheese contains less lactose than milk, and it is believed the friendly bacteria used to make yoghurt helps in the digestion of the lactose. It is quite possible therefore that one reason why some people develop lactose intolerance is because they no longer have enough of their own friendly bacteria to assist in its digestion.

12.3 Antibiotics

Your child may have true allergies to certain foods and you can test for these, however it may be that your child's digestive system needs some support and healing so that the digestive process improves and fewer protein molecules are able to pass through the gut lining and interact with the immune system and brain.

I mentioned earlier that certain substances can damage the delicate lining of our digestive systems and none more so than antibiotics.

Antibiotics indirectly have a negative influence on the health of our gut lining. Antibiotics are given to kill bacteria, they not only kill the bad ones that cause infection and illness but they also kill the good ones too.

I've already told you what an important role the good bacteria play so killing them off is not a good idea.

Unfortunately many children by the age of 10 have had several courses of antibiotics for various infections and so it is very likely that the health of their digestive tract is already quite impaired.

12.4 Candida

Reduced numbers of good bacteria in the gut, means the bad bacteria that also live there can begin to thrive. It also means that other undesirables like yeasts and parasites could take hold and multiply.

Too many of these and obvious digestive symptoms like bloating, wind, diarrhoea or constipation and foul smelling poo can appear. But there are other symptoms which you might not connect with the digestive system such as aching joints, brain fogginess and poor memory, persistent thrush and extreme tiredness.

One of the most common consequences of a disrupted balance in gut bacteria is something called candida. It is an overgrowth of a yeast that under normal circumstances lives in low levels in the gut but when the good bacteria diminish in numbers, this candida can multiply and grow very rapidly indeed.

Yeasts like candida feed off sugar and so a diet high in sugar will further encourage its growth.

Of the children I help that have learning difficulties, 45% of the parents reported candida in one or both parents. Children born to parents who are suffering from this condition do seem to have a greater risk of having problems.

Unlike the friendly gut bacteria that release substances to encourage the health and well being of the intestinal lining, the unfriendly bacteria along with any unfriendly yeasts like candida release substances that are actually quite toxic and damaging to the gut lining.

Again, this irritates and damages the gut lining and opens up the potential for undigested proteins to pass into the blood stream and even potentially reach the brain.

These toxic substances themselves also get absorbed into the blood stream and can lead to a wide variety of problems. In fact an unknown number of potential neurotoxins (toxins that affect the nervous system and brain) are released by unfriendly or abnormal gut bacteria.

So here again is another good reason to eat less sugar, eat more fibre and vegetables and drink more water to keep the digestive system healthy.

There are many things that can be done to help someone recover from a candida overgrowth and this will involve changes to the diet and quite possibly several courses of different supplements. It is always best to seek the advice of a qualified nutritional therapist when dealing with children.

Sixty per cent of my patients with learning difficulties have parents with family history of allergies, candida or learning difficulties.

Children with learning difficulties therefore are already most likely challenged by having parents in suboptimum health. Nutrient deficiencies, candida and allergies can all be passed from the parents to the child. So they will most likely have suboptimum health themselves and will react to well known offensive foods (or antinutrients).

Take my family. My father is dyscalculate with no concept of time. My sister and I were dyscalculate. My son was dyslexic. My father has food intolerances, I have had some brushes with that, and we have avoided the things that upset my father, in our son.

Family history plays a big part. But that doesn't mean there's nothing that can be done.

Knowledge about what makes you ill, can let you avoid those things until you recover or not.

12.5 Junk Foods

Since the 1950's scientists, chemists and food technologists have been inventing all manner of new ingredients and substances to enable food to be cost effectively mass produced whilst at the same time satisfying the taste buds and visual perception of the public who will buy that food.

They've invented preservatives, thickeners, stabilisers, acidity regulators, emulsifiers, colourings, anticaking agents and flavour enhancers to name but a few. Not to mention the pesticides and herbicides that are also widely used.

12.6 E Numbers

Our bodies are exposed to quite possibly hundreds of different chemicals on a daily basis, and many of them in or on our food. All food additives are given an E number to show that they have been assessed for safety and have been approved for use in food. Most substances however are only assessed and approved based on their individual effects and safety levels, there is very little data on the effects of consuming a combination of these additives on a regular basis, let alone over a lifetime.

To add to the confusion some E numbers are actually natural ingredients and pose no risk to health. There are other E numbers however that have been found to be quite detrimental to health. Recently many sweet manufactures have stopped using the harmful ones and are using natural ones.

Certain food additives have been linked to asthma, eczema, nettle rash, dermatitis, allergies, aggressive behaviour, hyperactivity, poor attention spans, poor impulse control, impaired memory and mental performance.

Sulphites, benzoates, tartrazine and other azodye colourings tend to be the most common culprits.

The UK Food Standards Agency recently commissioned a study by researchers at Southampton University into the effects of certain colours (sunset yellow (E110), quinoline yellow (E104), carmoisine (E122), allura red (E129), tartrazine (E102) and ponceau 4R (E124)) and the preservative sodium benzoate on children's behaviour. They found that the children's behaviour was worse with these additives in their diet than when they excluded, even in children with no previous history of hyperactive or disruptive behaviour.

In light of this research and a further study to confirm the results, the Food Standards Agency have requested a voluntary ban on the use of these colours and has requested manufacturers to find alternatives to these ingredients. Unfortunately without firm evidence of actual harm they are unable to ban the substances!

These colours are used in a number of soft drinks, sweets, cakes and ice cream. My advice is to steer clear of them, whether or not your child is hyperactive or not.

12.7 Zinc, mental health

The Food Standards Agency website (http://www.food.gov.uk) is keeping an updated list of products that do not contain the six food colourings associated with hyperactive behaviour. Another good reason for this is that another scientific study has looked into the effects of tartrazine (E102, the colour that makes drinks orangey-yellow) on mineral levels in the body. The scientists measured the amount of zinc in children's urine before and after the drink. What they found was that the drink containing E102 made the children excrete zinc. Zinc is one of the most essential nutrients for mental health and several studies have found a link between zinc deficiency and hyperactivity, learning and eating disorders.

Karen says: Zinc is such an important nutrient for developing children and to discover excretion of it is increased after consuming E102 colouring proves that the colouring is highly likely to be detrimental to health. Any substance that encourages the excretion or blocks the action of beneficial nutrients is called an antinutrient.

But that is a snapshot of one additive on one occasion. E102 is just one example of an antinutrient.

Children rarely just have one additive once. Many children are possibly having ten or more a day every day.

They are therefore highly likely to be deficient in most vitamins and minerals as well as essential fatty acids and protein.

That is why your child should avoid artificially created additives to food. The colourings flavourings, preservatives, monosodiumglutamate, nitrates, sweeteners and so on.

Let me give you an example. And you probably know a child like this. They have brown rings under their eyes, a crease across the bridge of their nose, they are irritable, very thirsty all the time, and crave sugar.

This child has food allergies (brown rings and nose crease), essential fat deficiency (thirst), and chromium deficiency (sugar craving and irritability).

Add that to brain wiring problems and you have a child who is unlikely to be happy and learning. If your child has learning problems or suffers from allergies or other health problems avoiding unnecessary food additives is a must.

There are two very useful books that every parent should have. The first is "E for Additives" by Maurice Hanssen, this book will tell you everything you need to know about every E number.

The other is the "Foresight Index Number Decoder". This is a little booklet available from a preconceptual care charity in the UK called Foresight (http://www.foresightpreconception. org.uk). It is a useful handbag sized guide to additives, colour coded for those to avoid and those that are safe.

It's not just artificial additives that can make children react. The Hyperactive Children's Support Group (http:// www.hacsg.org.uk) has a great deal of information on this. Common natural offenders are chocolate, nuts, cheeses, and chicken.

Reactions to substances in our foods can vary enormously. Some children react and others do not. Some have clear physical or mental symptoms like allergies or aggressive behaviour whilst in others symptoms can be mild and seemingly unconnected.

In case I haven't made it clear yet, feed your child a natural diet. Lots of vegetables, some meat, some oily fish, some fruit, lots of wild rice, brown rice and lentils, some potatoes, lots of water, some nuts and seeds. Keep it fresh, unprocessed and enjoy it.

This food will produce strong, robust children that will be ill less. Full happy tummies facilitate learning too.

I grow vegetables in my vegetable patch. Sometimes I start them off under cover. The plants that have enough water, soil borne nutrients and sunlight, survive well. Those starved of any of those, usually die.

They never make strong robust plants that produce a healthy crop. People are no different.

TAKE NOTE: drink more water, eat well, and get outside for some exercise and sunshine.

© Copyright Sue Cook and Karen Stevenson 2009

Further Reading
Dept W., The Hyperactive Children's Support Group, 71 Whyke lane, Chichester, West
Sussex PO19 7PD HACSG
hacsg@hacsg.org.uk
****

Further Research into Diets:
Feingold Diet
GAPS

More books in the series

Here is a free first chapter of some of the other books in the series. To get the book go to Amazon and type in Brainbuzzz (one word 3 Z) in the book section and a list of my books come up. Select from there.

First Chapter from my book on Lefthanders

LEFTHANDERS

Lefthandedness only affects about ten per cent of the population directly but it actually affects more than that. If there is a leftie in a family, then the whole family needs to be aware of what life is like for that person.

Or if you have a child who is a leftie, you need to understand them better too. I do know what it feels to have a child with learning difficulties, and I do know what it is like to help them. I hope you find the following interesting....

Left handers are not wrong. We are just different. Accept it. In my family growing up, there were two lefties and two righties. My mother and I are the left handers. It was a democratic household.

We had left handed scissors and right handed scissors. Nobody was teased for being the odd one out. Our differences were appreciated and discussed, not mocked. I have been laughed at by righties, and called Cack handed. Cack is not a pleasant insult.

And all because the brain is wired differently.
Odd isn't it? That is not acceptable to me, that people are verbally abused because of what boils down to ignorance.
I am probably one of the lucky ones, having grown up in a democratically handed household. But for many children, they are misunderstood, blamed, insulted, and not catered for. And that is ten per cent of the population.
If I say to you now 'lefthanders are different and have different needs' how do you react? If you are a right hander you might be thinking that this is nonsense and a stupid comment. But imagine being on the receiving end of that negativity when you do have genuinely different needs….
When my friends find out that I have left handed cooking equipment and left handed knives, and scissors, and rulers, they laugh. It is a total mystery that anyone should need such bizarre things.
But they have them automatically as a right hander, and do not even realise it. Everything we buy has been designed by someone, and where relevant, it is designed to be used by a right hander. So therefore it penalises the lefty. Accidentally.
I'm really hoping the Science Museum does a left hander room one day so the righties can try everything out and see for themselves what life through the looking glass is like. Cartons of milk are right handed (try pouring them with your left hand and you will see what I mean).
I have a left handed corkscrew and all the right handers cut themselves on it, so I have stopped using it. My friends cut themselves on my knives too, even when I warn them, they still cut themselves.
This is not meant to be a moan, rather an explanation of the hidden difficulties we have. Injuries and insults as well as awkwardness.
When I was at university I wrote a literature review on handedness and intelligence. I wanted to know if we really were stupid as lefthanders as we were so often told. I found out that we are not, we are often

more intelligent than righties, except if we have
brain damage.
So, aside from the scissors and knives, and injury
potential, I like being lefthanded. So do my leftie
friends.
We make the best of it. We feel it gives us an edge;
we think differently, we come to different
conclusions, we are far from ordinary. And I will
explain why.
Left handers differ from right handers more than just
by writing with the other hand.
There are two hemispheres, or sides, in the brain.
Right handers have a left hemisphere that is
dominant, in most cases, and left handers have a
dominant right hemisphere in most cases.
Each hemisphere does slightly different things from
the other, like non identical twins perhaps. So that
means that left handers do not think in the same way
as right handers, and they most certainly learn differently.

First Chapter On Being Dyscalculate in Maximise Your Child's
Potential

MY STORY
BEING DYSCALCULATE

(This was written in 2009, before I had been using neurodevelopment on myself. Now that I use neurodevelopment regularly, I can do some maths, though need to learn techniques so I know how to do it.)

There are not many books on this subject, or places where people can find out more about this. Much has been written on being dyslexic, but not on being dyscalculate. And information about this, is not written by someone who experiences the symptoms. I am aiming to address that, so that parents and other people with dyscalculia can have some 'aha' moments and begin to understand the experience a little better.

So what's it like?

The aim is to explain from a personal viewpoint what it is like to be dyscalculate, what the symptoms are, what is happening in the brain, and what to do about it.

Here is an introduction I wrote a couple of years ago.

'So I can't add up.

I can't look up something in the index of a book and remember the number long enough to find the page.

I can't learn to do maths

I can't work out how to do things with numbers.

I can't compare prices of things in supermarkets.

Even when I'm repeatedly told how to work maths things out, I can't remember it.

It's a nuisance. My school teachers shouted at me because they couldn't believe I didn't understand what they were trying to teach. Why can't an other wise bright girl do such a simple thing?

What we didn't know back then was that I couldn't do maths because I am dyscalculate. So is my Dad and my sister and I'm not too sure about Mum.

Being left handed doesn't help either because our eyes naturally scan from right to left. With words it is ok because the brain knows them so well, there is familiarity, though occasionally I have transposed parts of a word. For years I thought vitamin B6 was called Pyroxidine, not pyridoxine.

But with numbers, there is no consistency, they can be anything, so I usually transpose them or just get them in the wrong order. Numbers are a total mystery. I am told there are patterns to numbers and that they are logical. Numbers to me are like a foreign language that I have never been able to translate. I cannot decode it.I have helped children with dyscalculia and they have improved.

One such girl had an assessment done at a dyslexia establishment, and was told by the assessor, whom the mother was paying hundreds of pounds, that 'he had heard of dyscalculia but didn't know what it was'.

When my father was working at a dyslexia establishment he asked his colleagues about dyscalculia and was told 'just get them to check their work'.

These are unsatisfactory responses that demonstrate how little is understood of the maths equivalent to dyslexia. I have lived with this all my life. I slipped through the net at school for various reasons, among them the fact that dyslexia was unrecognised until I was about 12 and dyscalculia didn't even have a name.

So how do I cope? I spent years avoiding numbers. From when I left school to when I was a magazine editor and had to work out authors payments per word, I totally avoided them.

To me maths was more frightening than any monster. Being faced with a maths problem was enough to reduce me to tears. That is because my teachers made me like that by shouting at me.

It is very important when dealing with children with these problems that we accept them for who they are. They do not choose these problems but are forced to live with them. We as parents can facilitate their growth with patience, understanding, acceptance and love.

I know how hard it is. I have learning difficulties and am a parent of such a child and a daughter of someone who had them too.

This is why I am SO driven to help others. THERE ARE ANSWERS. (The brainbuzzz programme provides you with what you need.)

I remember my first day at school, the teacher was doing simple sums on the board. It was a total mystery to me. I could not understand how everyone could work out that this symbol 'add' this other symbol 'equalled' another symbol. Mystery.

And telling the time (which I finally mastered at the age of ten) was another mystery for a while too.

MY SYMPTOMS

I have the following symptoms:

• Inability to hold numbers in the brain for any length of time if there has to be something done to the number (this is because the information has to change hemispheres and to add just two numbers, the information must change hemispheres nine times (Sally Goddard's book The ABC of Learning explains this). So if the corpus callosum is insufficiently wired, the numbers fall off a cliff.)

• If I am remembering a number, then after a couple of minutes, the number slides to another number and I get confused. I no longer know what the original number was. Short term memory for numbers.

• Difficulty remembering formulae for mathematical processes. Confusion when recalling numbers.

• Difficulty remembering the meaning of the terms, such as decimal or fraction.

• Difficulty remembering where north south east and west are (I just have trouble with west).

• A dyscalculate person may be good at other academic subjects, but poor in maths (like me).

• Late development of any mathematical aptitude. Faulty processing of numbers.

• Difficulty understanding what is expected in a mathematical task.

• Acquired symptoms I have developed include: switching off when discussions of numbers occur, or anything to do with number processing.

• A feeling of panic if I am expected to perform any maths task. I switch off because I get lost immediately and I know that most of the time I will not be able to get any further on in the task, and it's no good getting cross with me about this. That is not going to help.

• Other symptoms I have include really sensitive hearing. Close loud noises really hurt my ears but do not hurt the ears of others. I do not seem to have three dimensional (directional hearing). I have never been able to tell where a sound comes from. My eyes are very sensitive to the light and I need dark glasses outside, in my case this is due to Irlen Syndrome.

HOW DO THESE SYMPTOMS AFFECT A PERSON'S LIFE?

School is going to be the first place where the torture of maths will be felt. For me it was pure torture being expected to be able to do adding up when I didn't even know what the symbols were, that represented quantities (these are known as numbers). Numbers are a code. No one explained the code and it took me a long time to work it out for myself. Non-dyscalculate people I am told, just understand this, whereas I did not.

Assuming knowledge in a child is an area where we need to take care. Not all children's brains mature at the same rate and not all are school ready at four years old when they start school in the UK. Neurodevelopmentalists have noticed that when a child's adult front teeth emerge, they are ready to read. There are of course exceptions, I have seen this myself, but as a general rule of thumb, children with earlier dentition tend to read earlier. My adult front teeth came in quite late at eight and !5

a half. My older son was even later. I couldn't read before I was eight (but I made up for it with gusto).

A child with a brain immaturity, lateness or dyscalculia, will be late achieving milestones, if at all.

As a child, I wanted to please, and do well. I was not being deliberately naughty by not being able to do maths, but teachers still thought it was ok to shout at me. That's not ok with me.

Such a child will probably always lag behind at school without knowledgeable intervention.

Failure at exam level is also likely. I failed maths O level three times and never achieved it.

Has it held me back in life? Yes, of course. Both the lack of maths qualification and not being able to perform maths, has been a stumbling block. But my attitude is that our stumbling blocks are best made into stepping stones; let's rise above it, learn from it and move on.

Comparing prices in supermarkets can be a tricky job when you can't remember the numbers you are trying compare (having converted them onto the same quantities; supermarkets price some comparable items in say Kilos and some in milligrams). I've got better at that. Looking up a number in the Yellow Pages was always difficult for me: I'd remember the first number; transpose the next two and forget the last. Then I worked out that if I said the number out loud, I could remember it long enough to find the page. Hearing it accessed a different part of my brain from seeing it.

Also as a left hander, my eyes naturally scan from right to left, thus the transposition of the letters, I do this occasionally with words, but it doesn't show as a problem because words can only be spelt one way and I know how to spell, so I don't mix my words up. Numbers can be in any order so are easier to make mistakes with.

It is not just straight numbers where the fault with brain shows. I have trouble processing certain concepts. I tried to learn astrology once, but could not remember the details. Whether a side effect of my brain issue, I have developed an extremely good memory, long term, short term, visual, detail and so on. I remember massive amounts and I surprise people with what I can recall. So when I struggle to get to grips with something, it annoys me, and these days I remember why; it's a processing difficulty using my maths brain.

For more information on how Sue Cook works with special needs including dyslexia, dyspraxia, dyscalculia, Aspergers, Autism, ADHD, mutism, ataxia, cerebral palsy, go to her website www.brainbuzzz.co.uk and note there are three Z.
Sue is on LinkedIn, Facebook, Pinterest, and so on and she invites you to connect.
Sue also trains people to become a neurodevelopment practitioner, and she sees patients.

20455886R00043

Printed in Great Britain
by Amazon